Allergy Busters

also by Kathleen A. Chara and Paul J. Chara, Jr.

Sensory Smarts
A Book for Kids with ADHD or Autism Spectrum Disorders Struggling with Sensory Integration Problems
Kathleen A. Chara and Paul J. Chara, Jr. with Christian P. Chara
Illustrated by J.M. Berns
ISBN 1 84310 783 X

of related interest

Can I tell you about Asperger Syndrome?
A Guide for Friends and Family
Jude Welton
Illustrated by Jane Telford
Foreword by Elizabeth Newson
ISBN 1 84310 206 4

A User Guide to the GF/CF Diet for Autism,
Asperger Syndrome and AD/HD
Luke Jackson
With appendices by Jacqui Jackson
Foreword by Marilyn Le Breton
ISBN 1 84310 055 X

Diet Intervention and Autism
Implementing the Gluten Free and Casein Free Diet for Autistic Children and Adults – A Practical Guide for Parents
Marilyn Le Breton
Foreword by Rosemary Kessick, Allergy Induced Autism
ISBN 1 85302 935 1

The AiA Gluten and Dairy Free Cookbook
Compiled by Marilyn Le Breton
Foreword by Rosemary Kessick, Allergy Induced Autism
ISBN 1 84310 067 3

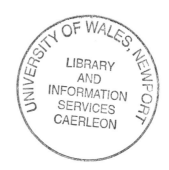

Allergy Busters

A Story for Children with Autism or Related Spectrum Disorders Struggling with Allergies

Kathleen A. Chara and Paul J. Chara, Jr. with Karston J. Chara

Illustrated by J.M. Berns

With gluten-free and casein-free recipes by Angela Litzinger

Jessica Kingsley Publishers
London and Philadelphia

First published in 2004
by Jessica Kingsley Publishers
116 Pentonville Road
London N1 9JB, UK
and
400 Market Street, Suite 400
Philadelphia, PA 19106, USA

www.jkp.com

Copyright © Kathleen A. Chara and Paul J. Chara Jr. 2004
Illustrations copyright © J.M. Berns 2004

Library of Congress Cataloging in Publication Data

Chara, Kathleen A. (Kathleen Ann), 1965-
    Allergy busters : a story for children with autism or related spectrum disorders struggling with allergies / Kathleen A. Chara, Paul J. Chara, Jr. and Karston J. Chara ; illustrated by J.M. Berns ; with gluten-free and casein-free recipes by Angela Litzinger.
                                          p. cm.
    ISBN 1-84310-782-1 (pbk.)
    1. Chara, Karston J. (Karston John), 1993---Mental health. 2. Autistic children--Biography. 3. Allergy in children--Juvenile literature. I. Chara, Paul J. (Paul John), 1953- II. Chara, Karston, J. (Karston John), 1993- III. Title.
    RJ506.A9C4353 2004
    618.92'85882--dc22
                                                        2004010961

British Library Cataloguing in Publication Data

A CIP catalogue record for this book is available from the British Library

ISBN 1 84310 782 1

Printed and Bound in Great Britain by
Athenaeum Press, Gateshead, Tyne and Wear

Contents

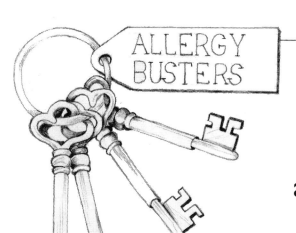

Introduction to Parents, Caregivers, and Professionals

Allergies can cause significant stress for the whole family, particularly for families who are already dealing with children on the autism spectrum. Children who suffer from allergies often have to miss out on fun-filled activities, such as school trips or birthday parties, leaving them feeling isolated and frustrated. Siblings of allergy sufferers may also become frustrated or angry because the family is not able to engage in certain activities or eat certain foods. And parents often feel overwhelmed in trying to meet the seemingly never-ending needs of their family. The aim of this book is to relieve stress on over-burdened families by providing a simple, yet effective, means to help children (and their families) to recognize and control allergies. The pages that follow are based on the real-life experiences of one young boy, Karston, who has struggled with sensory and visual problems, fine and gross motor delays, and especially from food and environmental allergies. In order to cope with the allergies, Karston and his parents developed a plan that has proved to be very effective. This plan is explained to the young child and gently encourages her or him to join a club called Allergy Busters by using the four Allergy Buster Keys. These keys are:

- recognize your allergies and avoid them
- take your medicine and vitamins
- be alert to allergy triggers
- creatively plan ahead for outings and special events.

A behavioral chart entitled the Allergy Buster Reward System and guidelines for using it are provided to assist families in following these four Allergy Buster Keys. Two certificates, one for the allergy sufferer and one for siblings, are also included. To encourage family fun, we have provided information and recipes for a gluten-free and casein-free pizza party (numerous resources are provided to buy or make these foods). A unique aspect of this book is that siblings of allergy sufferers also participate and receive a certificate for helping a sibling with allergies and thus become an Allergy Buster too! Many families have become Allergy Busters so come aboard and join the fun!!

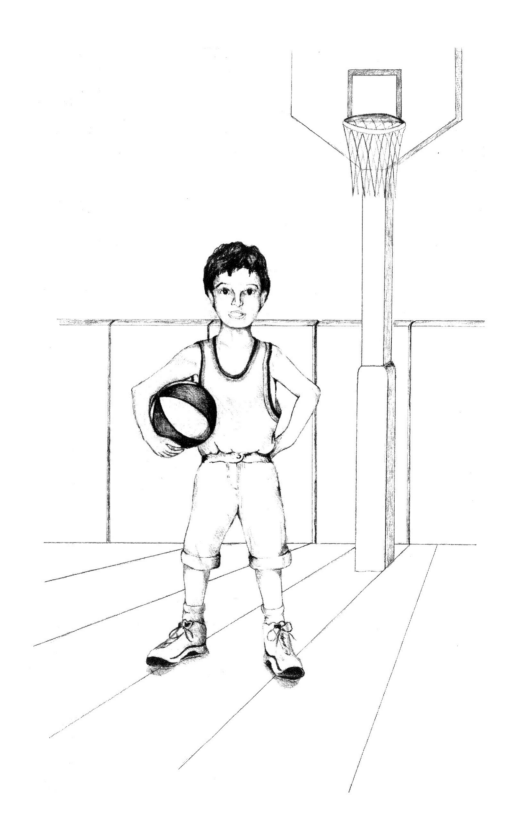

Allergy Busters

Hello! My name is Karston and I have allergies. Maybe you have allergies too or know someone who does. Allergies are a medical problem. This medical problem can cause a lot of other problems for children and their families. Having allergies means that there are certain things that you can't eat or be around. These things that you are allergic to are called allergens. Your body can't handle allergens like other people can. Allergies can be a real bummer and cause stress and frustrations for families—especially for kids like you and me.

There are two types of allergies: food allergies and environmental allergies. When you have food allergies, there are certain foods you should not eat because your body reacts badly to them. Common food allergies include peanuts, soy, chocolate, milk (especially casein) and wheat (especially gluten). Casein is a type of protein found in milk OR things that are made with milk, like cheese. Gluten is a sticky protein found in most wheat, barley, oats, or rye items, such as pizza, breads, rolls and bagels.

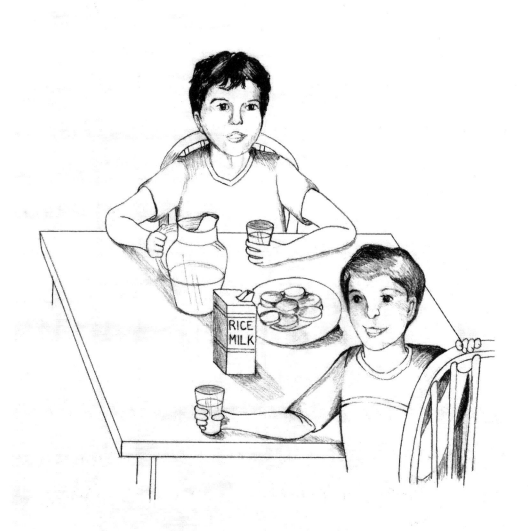

If you have environmental allergies, it means that there are things in the area that you live in that your body will react badly to, like grass, dust, bug bites, cats, rubber items, or mold. Sometimes I think I am allergic to my brothers, but my parents say that doesn't count! Oh well.

Some kids have only one type of allergy but some, like me, have both types. My main food allergies are to sugar and milk (casein), and my big environmental allergies are to dust and mold (the stuff that grows on some trees). What are you or someone you know allergic to? I used to think that refined sugar or milk was in everything. But, I found out that I was wrong.

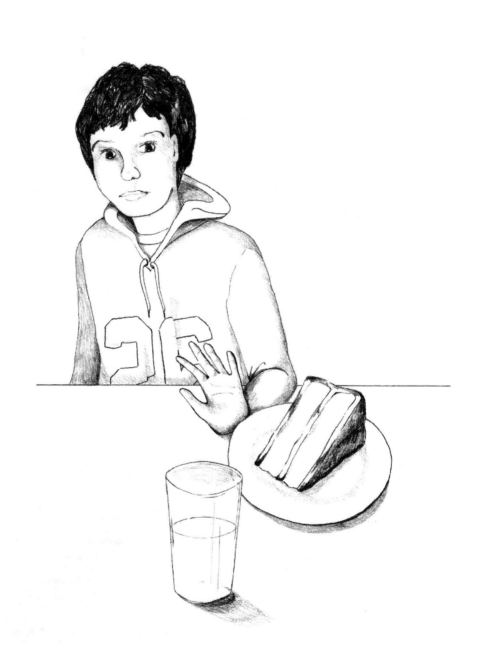

I also used to think I was the only kid who had all these allergies and had to say NO THANK YOU to things I liked. If you have allergies or just learned that you have allergies, remember you are NOT the only kid who has allergies. Lots of kids have allergies.

I have learned to still have lots of fun and to take care of my allergies. Let me tell you about my life with allergies.

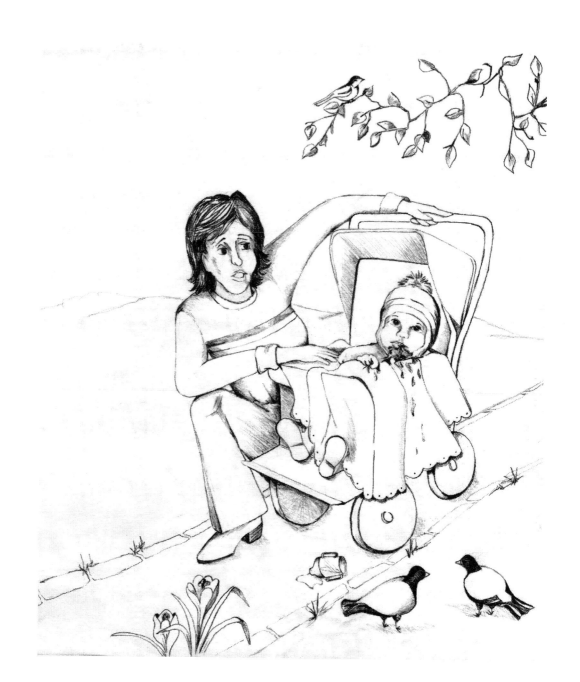

When I was born, my parents did not know that I had allergies. I was too little to talk, so I didn't tell them. My parents said that when I was born my skin was dry, cracked, and bleeding. YUCK! Later, we all learned that this is often a sign that a baby may grow up to have allergies.

My mom said that when I was a baby if my parents took me for a car ride in the country, I would usually throw up. DOUBLE YUCK!! Did your parents ever notice things that bothered you even as a baby? Maybe you should ask them about it.

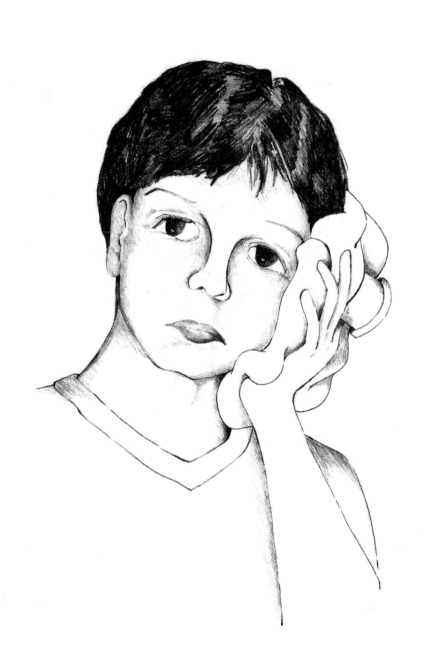

When I was three years old, I began getting sick every day. I remember one time when my mom gave me M&Ms and later I got a VERY BIG HEADACHE and VERY BAD STOMACH ACHE and we didn't know why. These big headaches are called migraines. I had these VERY BIG HEADACHES and STOMACH ACHES for the next year and a half—talk about a long year and a half!

All kids react differently to allergies. Some kids get a rash on their bodies, other kids get stomach aches, headaches, runny noses, repeated ear infections, diarrhea (my dad calls this the "soup butt"), or breathing problems. YUCK! Other kids get into bigger trouble when they have something they are allergic to. I know a little girl who wasn't growing or talking until she stopped eating foods with gluten in them. WOW! What happens to you when you eat or are around what you are allergic to?

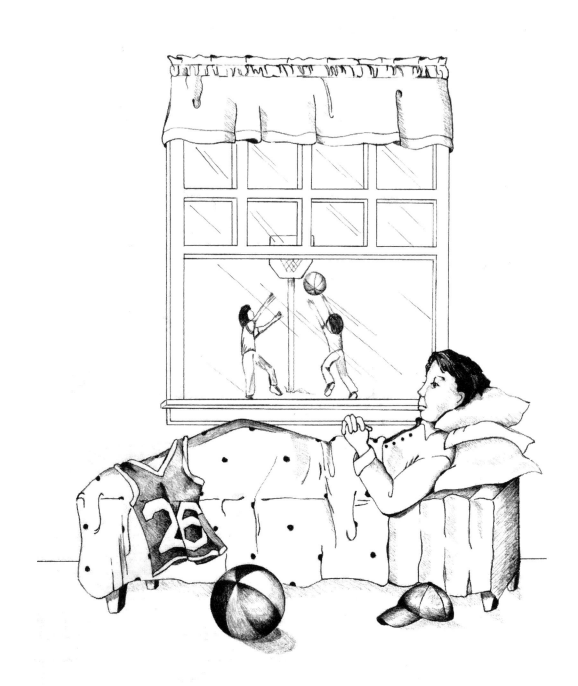

Being sick all the time was painful and annoying. I didn't feel good enough to do the things I liked to do, like ride my bike, play ball with my friends, or go to the park. I even missed my own birthday party once—what a bummer! How about you and your family? How have allergies affected your life?

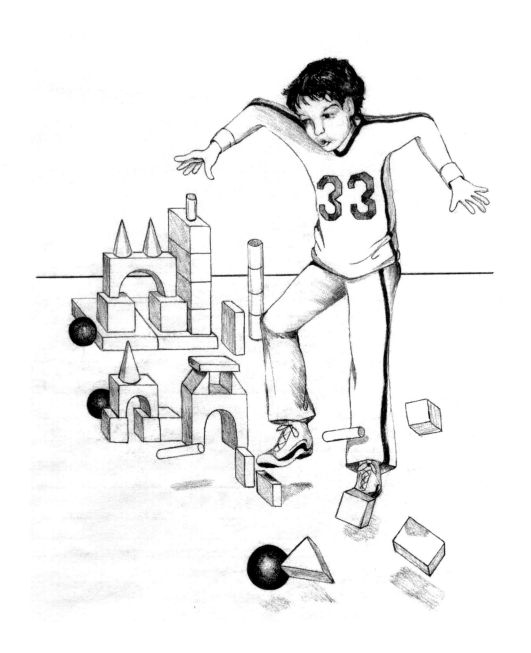

My family says that I am not very fun to be around when I am sick from my allergies. I can easily get frustrated and sometimes I get mean. It is just not much fun being sick from allergies. Is it hard for you to keep doing what you are supposed to do when you are having allergy problems? Sometimes, I find it hard to pay attention in school when I am not feeling well. Other times, I get really excited and like to run all over the place. Still other times, it seems like I have no energy at all and I just stay on the couch like a lumpy pillow. One thing that I have realized is that the other problems I am working on only get worse when I have eaten or have been around things I am allergic to. You may not like to admit it, but I bet the same is true for you too!

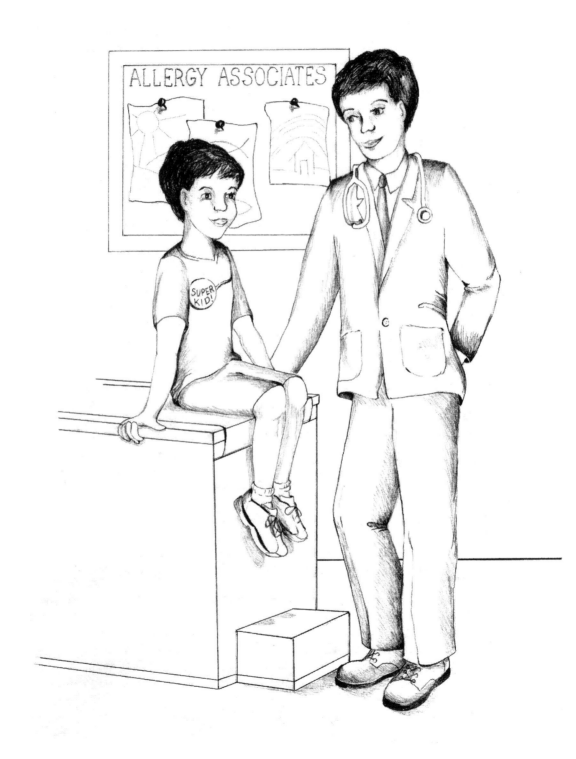

When I was five years old my parents took me to a big hospital called the Mayo Clinic for tests to see why I was sick all the time. We still did not know I was getting sick from allergies. The doctors said I had allergies. So I went to another place called Allergy Associates and had some more tests. These tests were a little like getting dozens of tiny needle shots. It hurt a little bit at first, but I didn't even cry! I even got a cool toy from my parents when the tests were done. I am glad I had these tests, though, because they told us what I was allergic to and I really wanted to stop getting sick and start having more fun again like the other kids my age.

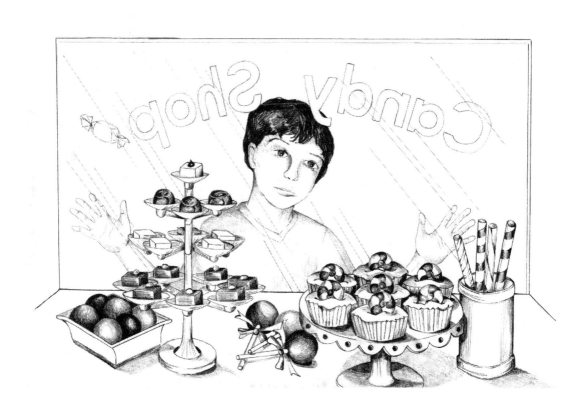

These tests told us that one thing I was allergic to was refined sugar or foods with corn syrup in them. I said, "WHAT? I LOVE CANDY! How is a growing boy to live without cotton candy, pop, cookies, and birthday cake with extra frosting?" I was not happy to hear about this! I thought my life was over—RUINED! I dreamt of having friends over for my birthday party and eating only green beans and carrots. I knew something had to be done—this was AWFUL!! Some of my friends can't have foods with gluten or milk in them, and they reacted the same way as I did: "WHAT? Everything has gluten or milk in it! Doesn't it?" But don't give up! I used to think that way too, but I now know about some great recipes that really do taste good. Your parents can look at and try tons of new recipes that are great to eat and are still foods you and I are not allergic to. You may have to try out a lot of ideas for new foods before you find the perfect recipe, but keep trying and tasting so that you can find the best ones for you. I did and so can you!! I put some ideas for a pizza party at the back of this book—just for YOU!

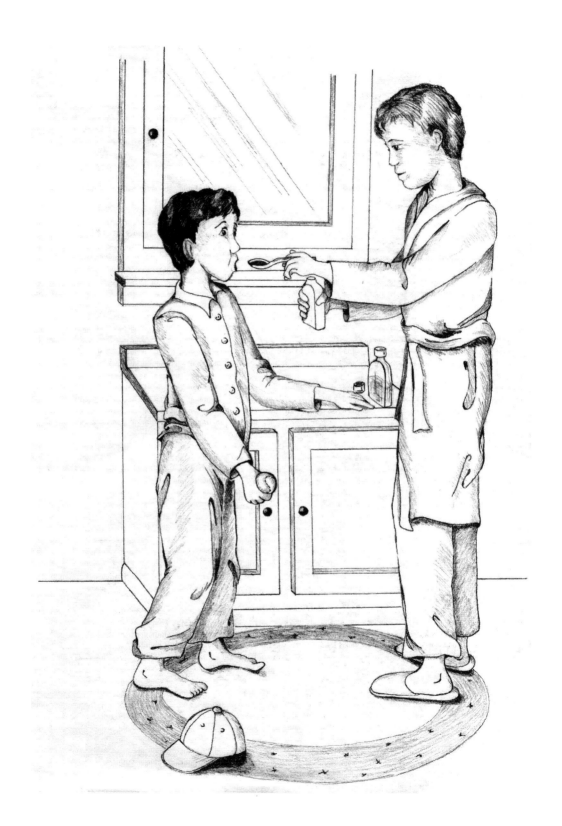

The tests also said I had to start taking medicine every day. Just think about it. First, I am told not to eat anything with milk or sugar, and then I hear about taking medicine every day. "WHAT? Here I am already taking vitamins and some medicines, and now I have to take more?" It's enough to make a grown boy cry! Sometimes, life just isn't fair: less of the stuff that tastes good and more of the stuff that tastes bad! SUPER DOUBLE YUCK!!!!

I now take medicines at night and in the morning to help with my allergies. Some kids have shots to help with their allergies. I take a small pill at night and use a nasal spray each morning and night. I also take small drops of the things I am allergic to, to help my body learn not to react badly to them. At first, I didn't want to start taking more medicines, especially every day. But now it's no big deal! How about you? Do you have to get shots, or take medicines, or stop eating certain foods? Do you know the names of your allergies and medicines or vitamins?

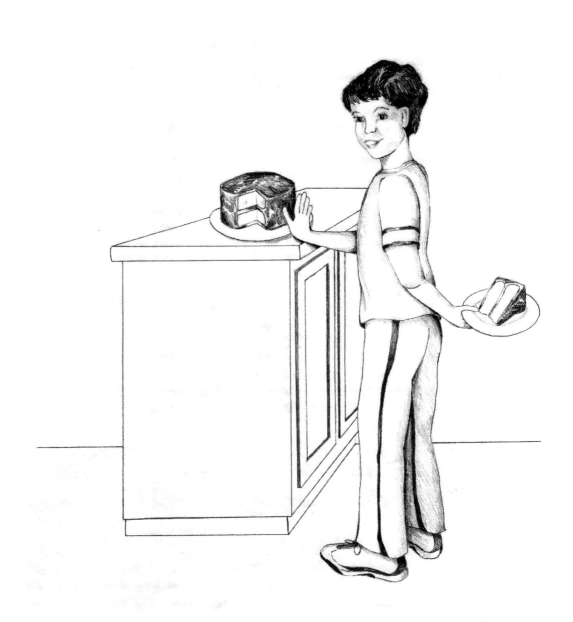

Well, I didn't like this allergy thing one bit, of course. I am sure you do not like having allergies either. Who would? I can't have the foods I really like and I have to take medicines EVERY DAY. This did not seem right or good to me and I decided to fight back. So, I came up with the "Karston Strikes Back" plan.

My plan was simple: I would just do what I had always done before. I pretended I did not have allergies, faked taking my medicines, snuck the foods I really wanted to eat, and played in places I knew would cause me trouble. But, there was ONE BIG PROBLEM. Although Mom and Dad did not catch on to all my tricks, my body knew. My plan of pretending and sneaking was not working because those VERY BIG HEADACHES and VERY BIG STOMACH ACHES always reminded me that I was not doing what I needed to do to take care of myself, my allergies, and my body. I needed to come up with a new plan—a plan that worked! I needed a plan that didn't have everyone mad at me for my behavior—a plan that still allowed me to have fun and friends.

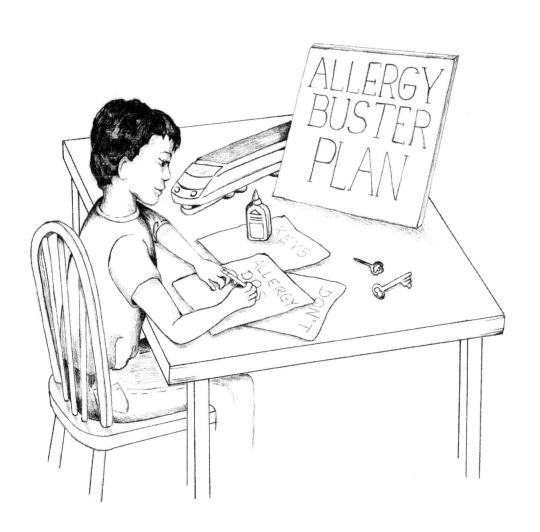

I thought I would tell you about my new plan to live with allergies, just in case your plan isn't working well either. I call this plan the Allergy Buster Plan. You and I can both use this plan to take control of our allergies. My Allergy Buster Plan has four important Allergy Buster Keys. I sure am glad I became an Allergy Buster. Would you like to join a group of kids called Allergy Busters too? Allergy Busters are kids who take control of their allergies by using the four Allergy Buster Keys and start having fun again without getting sick or hurting their bodies. Here are the four Allergy Buster Keys. I sure do hope you use these keys. I do and they help me out a lot. If you use these Allergy Buster Keys, then you will be an Allergy Buster too! Well, let's get going!

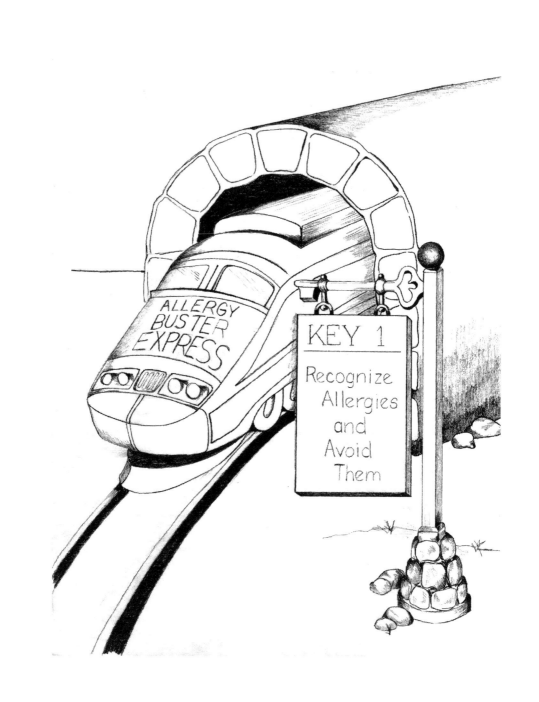

Allergy Buster Key #1

RECOGNIZE your allergies and **AVOID** them. It is very important to stay away from what causes allergies and to not eat what you are allergic to. Allergy Busters can say what they are allergic to and what they will do to avoid their allergies. Try to fill in this sentence: "I am allergic to _____, so I stay away from it by _____ _____."

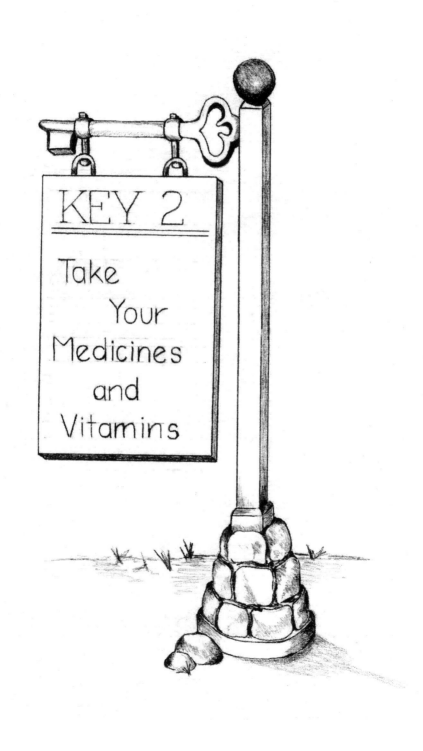

Allergy Buster Key #2

TAKE your **MEDICINES** and **VITAMINS** even if you do not want to. I know this stuff can sometimes taste bad and be a real pain, especially when you are tired or in a hurry. But just remember, allergies are a much bigger pain! Allergy Busters know the name of their medicines and take them, just like the doctor wants us to—**NO MATTER WHAT**! Allergy Busters have learned that doctors and parents are smart and care tons about us. We know that when we stop our medicines or don't take them on time we hurt our bodies. So, we take all of our medicines **ON TIME**. Allergy Busters say: "I, _____ (your name), will take my medicines and vitamins on time."

Allergy Buster Key #3

Be **ALERT** to allergy triggers. Allergy Busters learn to say **NO THANK YOU** to things we are allergic to. **BEFORE** we go places, we ask questions to find out if the places are allergy-safe. **BEFORE** we eat food, we ask questions to find out if the foods are allergy-safe. Think of your allergies as being hidden, but you, as an Allergy Buster are like a detective, finding out what you are allergic to and avoiding it. Allergy Busters can learn to read food labels and recognize how one allergen may have many different names on food labels. Allergy Busters can say: "No thank you, I am allergic to _____, may I do or have something else?"

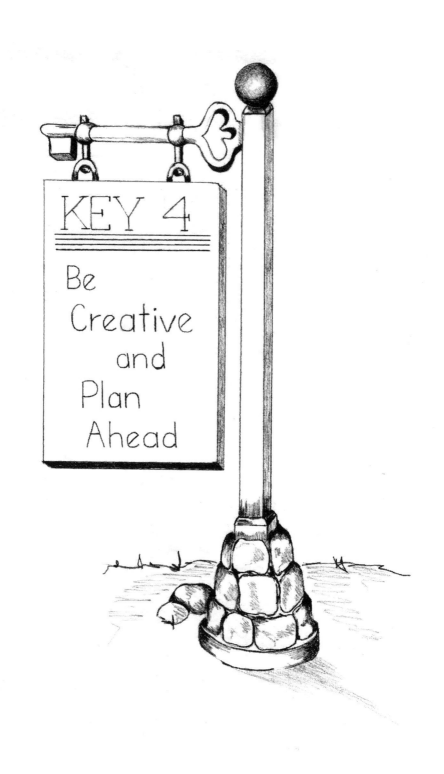

Allergy Buster Key #4

Creatively PLAN AHEAD for outings and special events. We think ahead if allergies may be a problem where we are going to be, like a birthday party, sleep over, or at our favorite camp. Allergy Busters bring needed items to use, such as allergy medicine, or allergy-safe foods to eat to replace the stuff we are allergic to. This way we can have just as much fun as everyone else—maybe even more if we bring enough for friends too! Parents can help too by checking to see what will be on the menu of places we may go. Allergy Busters are not afraid to try new foods, find new places to play, and love different animals. Try to fill in this statement: "I will take _____ with me on outings and I will try _____ three times before I decide whether I like it or not."

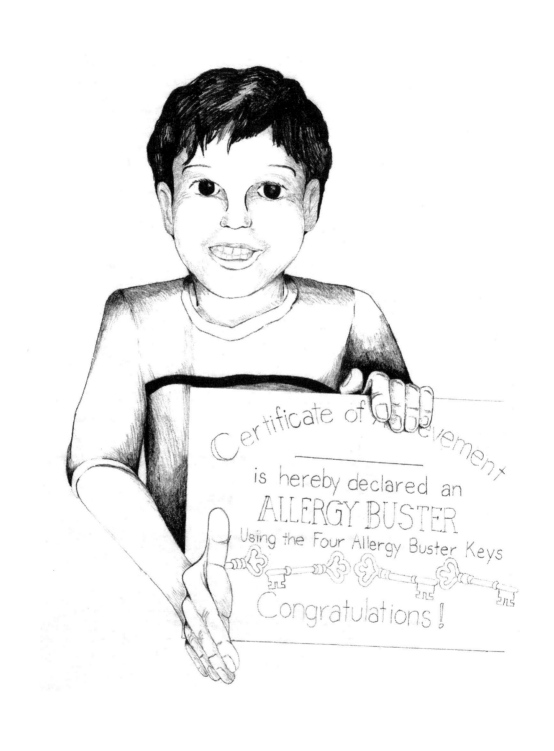

Do you want to use these four Allergy Buster Keys? Well, if so, then, CONGRATULATIONS!! You are now an Allergy Buster too! And, to properly congratulate you, I made a certificate for you and your family to fill out! Maybe you and your family will agree on a small prize for being an Allergy Buster by following the four Allergy Buster Keys. Remember, Allergy Busters recognize and avoid their allergies, take their medicines and vitamins, are alert to allergy triggers, and creatively plan ahead to bring extras for special outings. Remember, Allergy Busters need to learn how to read food labels as soon as they can.

Certificate of Achievement

_____

is hereby declared an

ALLERGY BUSTER

by Using the Four Allergy Buster Keys

1 RECOGNIZE ALLERGIES AND AVOID THEM

2 TAKE YOUR MEDICINES AND VITAMINS

3 BE ALERT

4 BE CREATIVE AND PLAN AHEAD

Congratulations!

_____
CHILD

_____
PARENT / PROFESSIONAL

Karsten
PRESIDENT

Certificate of Achievement

is hereby declared an

ALLERGY BUSTER HELPER

by Using the Four Allergy Buster Keys

1 RECOGNIZE ALLERGIES AND AVOID THEM

2 TAKE YOUR MEDICINES AND VITAMINS

3 BE ALERT

4 BE CREATIVE AND PLAN AHEAD

Congratulations !

Karston
PRESIDENT

CHILD

PARENT / PROFESSIONAL

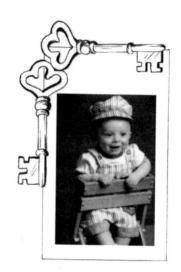

Now I am ten years old and I have had allergies for a long time and I've been on medicine since I was five. I sometimes still get that VERY BIG HEADACHE, but a lot less now that I follow my Allergy Buster Keys. There are lots of kids like us who have allergies and still have tons of fun in life. I love to ride my bike, play sports with my brothers and friends, and do weights with my dad. I have learned to take care of my allergies, to be happy, and to have tons of fun. So can you! Remember, always be an Allergy Buster and tell other kids about our four Allergy Buster Keys so they can have fun like us!

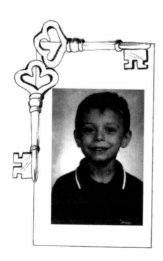

Your friend,

Karston

Karston, aka Allergy Buster

Allergy Buster Reward System

Guidelines for developing an effective reward system

The word *reward* is basically synonymous with the psychological term *reinforcement*. Psychologists define reinforcement as any stimulus (an event or object) that increases the likelihood of a particular behavior. A reward can be a powerful tool for increasing the frequency of desirable behaviors. However, a century of psychological research has demonstrated that the effectiveness of using a reward system is greatly affected by how it is set up and how it is implemented. To help you maximize the effectiveness of your reward system, we offer the following guidelines, organized around three basic steps.

1. Identify the behaviors you want to change.
2. Determine what to use as a reward.
3. Aim for long-term success.

Step 1: Identify the behaviors you want to change

A. DETERMINE THE IMPORTANCE OF BEHAVIORS

Rank behaviors in order from most important (e.g., taking medication) to least important (e.g., wiping nose on sleeve).

B. DETERMINE THE EASE OF CHANGING BEHAVIORS

Rank behaviors in order from easiest for the child to change (e.g., taking vitamins) to hardest for the child to change (e.g., refusing an offer of a desirable food that is also an allergy trigger).

C. DETERMINE FREQUENCY OF BEHAVIORS

Rank behaviors in order from most frequent (e.g., complains a lot) to least frequent (e.g., rarely eats fruit).

Step 2: Determine what to use as a reward

A. TWO BASIC WAYS OF REWARDING BEHAVIOR

1. *Reward training.* If the child acceptably performs a desired behavior, a reward is given.

2. *Omission training.* If the child stops (or decreases to an acceptable level) an undesired behavior, a reward is given.

B. WHAT MAKES A GOOD REWARD?

1. *The matching principle.* The frequency of behavior will be affected by how much children value a particular reward. A reward that has little value to children will have little impact in changing their behavior. Ask the child to give you examples of what he or she thinks is a good reward. Then, within reasonable limits, negotiate with the child what the reward(s) will be.

2. *Salience.* Children will change their behavior to get a reward that has a high value to them. However, if the value is too high, once the reward is stopped or greatly lessened, the behavior changed by the reward will revert to its pre-reward frequency. If the value of the reward is not too high, then even if the reward is stopped or greatly lessened, the rewarded behavior is likely to maintain its rewarded frequency and not revert to its pre-reward rate of occurrence. For example, one child is given 20 gold coins for every book that is read, whereas another child is given only one small silver coin for each book that is read. The monetary rewards are then terminated for each child. The child rewarded with the 20 gold coins is most likely to greatly decrease the time spent reading books or to stop reading. However, the child given the smaller reward is likely to continue reading at the rate that was rewarded. Simply put, rewards that are too valuable lower the probability that a child will continue a behavior—after the reward for it is removed—for its own sake.

3. *The Premack principle*. Anything that a child does frequently can be used to reward something that the child does infrequently. For example, J.J. loves to watch television but hates to eat vegetables. J.J. is then put on a reward schedule where every time a certain amount of veggies are eaten, a certain amount of television viewing is gained. In other words, viewing television is made to be dependent on eating veggies.

4. *The token economy*. A token is something that is used to represent a reward. In a token economy, children earn tokens that are eventually redeemed for monetary rewards or other desirable activities/objects. For example, a plus (+) is used to represent a certain amount of money. A child is then told that plusses will be given for specific behaviors that the child performs. At the end of a specified time, the plusses are counted and then exchanged for money. Most token economies include "reverse rewards" which can decrease the amount of tokens earned. Thus, good behaviors earn plusses and bad behaviors earn minuses, which reduce the number of plusses. Using "reverse rewards" provides consequences for undesirable behaviors and can increase the incentive for the child to perform desired behaviors—the child works extra hard to make up for the loss of plusses. However, if too many minuses are given, a child may lose the incentive to stick with the reward system. A token economy can provide a sense of immediate reward for the child (making the reward more effective) while delaying the administration of the actual reward (who wants to carry around a bag of coins in order to reward the child every time an acceptable behavior is performed?). Many children prefer stickers instead of plusses. Another approach is to have different levels of achievement: red = 1 reward; yellow = 2 rewards; green = 3 rewards; blue = 4 rewards.

Step 3: Aim for long-term success

A. START SMALL

1. Begin rewarding behaviors that are least important and easiest to change (see Step 1, A and B).

2. Begin using small amounts of rewards for these initial behaviors.

B. SHAPING

1. Gradually work in more difficult behaviors to change (see Step 1, A and C).

2. Gradually increase the amount of rewards used: the more difficult and/or more important the behavior, the greater the amount of reward used to modify it (but keep in mind Step 2, B2).

C. KEYS TO LONG-TERM SUCCESS

1. *Consistency.* Once a reward system is begun, stick to it! If a day or more is missed, don't despair, just get back to the system. The greater the consistency in using the reward system, the greater the likelihood of long-term success in developing positive behaviors.

2. *Attitude.* Make the reward system fun for the child! Deemphasize the failures and accentuate the successes. Give the child frequent feedback about how successful she or he has been, and encourage the child toward future successes.

3. *Frequency.* The more often and longer you use the reward system, the greater the likelihood that the rewarded behaviors will be permanently changed for the better! The reward system is helping children learn constructive habits, habits that are likely to be continued throughout their lives—even after the reward system is no longer used.

Suggested goals are given in the chart below. A blank chart to fill in yourself appears on the next page.

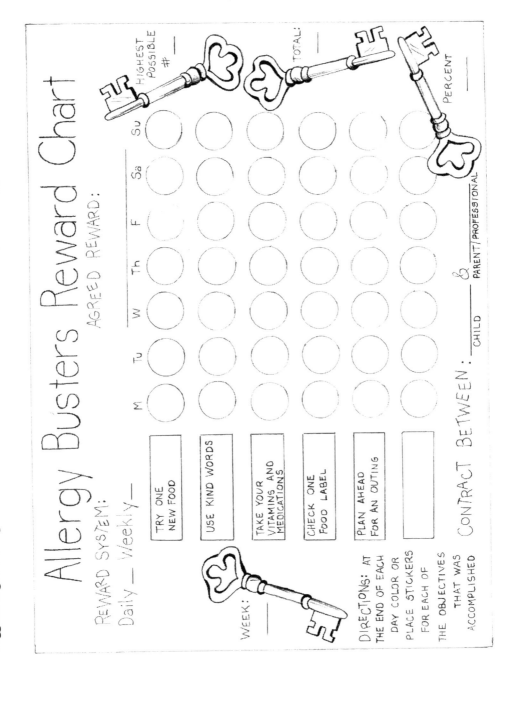

Allergy Busters Reward Chart

REWARD SYSTEM:
Daily — Weekly —

AGREED REWARD: _____

	M	Tu	W	Th	F	Sa	Su
TRY ONE NEW FOOD	◯	◯	◯	◯	◯	◯	◯
USE KIND WORDS	◯	◯	◯	◯	◯	◯	◯
TAKE YOUR VITAMINS AND MEDICATIONS	◯	◯	◯	◯	◯	◯	◯
CHECK ONE FOOD LABEL	◯	◯	◯	◯	◯	◯	◯
PLAN AHEAD FOR AN OUTING	◯	◯	◯	◯	◯	◯	◯
	◯	◯	◯	◯	◯	◯	◯

HIGHEST POSSIBLE # _____

TOTAL: _____

PERCENT _____

WEEK: _____

DIRECTIONS: AT THE END OF EACH DAY COLOR OR PLACE STICKERS FOR EACH OF THE OBJECTIVES THAT WAS ACCOMPLISHED

CONTRACT BETWEEN: _____ CHILD & _____ PARENT/PROFESSIONAL

Allergy Busters Reward Chart

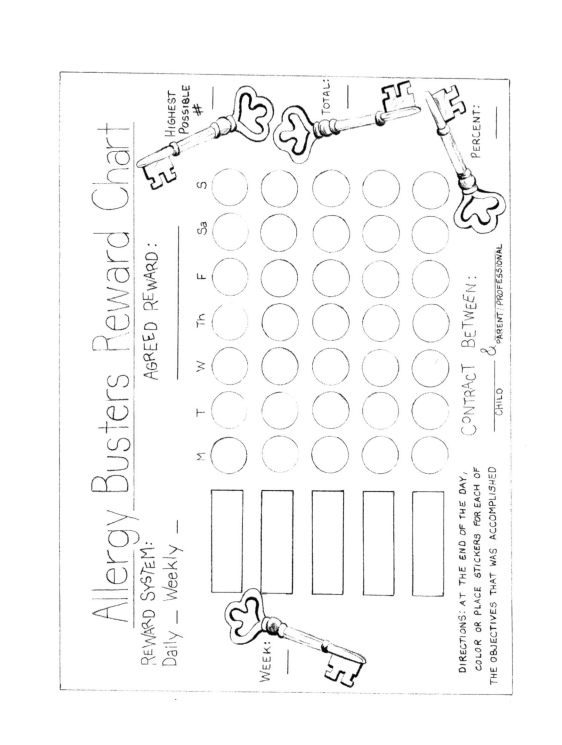

REWARD SYSTEM:
Daily — Weekly —

AGREED REWARD:

HIGHEST
POSSIBLE
#

	M	T	W	Th	F	Sa	S
	◯	◯	◯	◯	◯	◯	◯
	◯	◯	◯	◯	◯	◯	◯
	◯	◯	◯	◯	◯	◯	◯
	◯	◯	◯	◯	◯	◯	◯
	◯	◯	◯	◯	◯	◯	◯

TOTAL: ____

PERCENT: ____

WEEK: ____

CONTRACT BETWEEN:

____ & ____
CHILD   PARENT / PROFESSIONAL

DIRECTIONS: AT THE END OF THE DAY,
COLOR OR PLACE STICKERS FOR EACH OF
THE OBJECTIVES THAT WAS ACCOMPLISHED

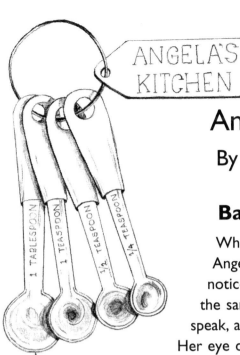

ANGELA'S KITCHEN

Angela's Kitchen

By Angela Litzinger

Background

When their daughter Eliana was one year old, Angela Litzinger and her husband Tim began to notice that she didn't seem to be developing in the same way as her elder brother. She didn't speak, and she didn't seem to respond to sound. Her eye contact was very erratic. She didn't walk until nearly 18 months. Eliana was short, very thin, and had many developmental delays. Shortly after her third birthday, after years of medical testing, Angela and Tim were told that their daughter had celiac disease, a destruction of the villi in the small intestine caused by intolerance to gluten. They decided to remove as much gluten as possible from her diet and the results were amazing! Their daughter grew over three inches in three months. Her hair, always very thin and wispy, started to thicken and grow. She slept through the night for the first time in her life as her apnea and snoring stopped. Her language and social skills, especially her eye contact, improved dramatically. Eliana now is in a kindergarten class, active with her many friends at school and Sunday school, and takes swimming and sport classes at the YMCA.

However, when accidentally exposed to gluten she will become very confused and inarticulate. Dark circles will form under her eyes, sleep will be troubled, and diarrhea problems will begin. To avoid this, Angela makes most of her meals at home. The following recipes are from Angela's kitchen. She hopes you will enjoy them and try them with your own children. The family that cooks together gets messy and laughs together!!

Party Recipes

To eat

These recipes are free of dairy products, gluten, refined sugar, corn, and soy.

GF/CF PIZZA

Pizza is a "must have" for kids. Unlike most GF/CF crusts that must be scooped and shaped with a spatula and moistened hands, you can knead and shape this dough making it more like gluten dough and more kid-friendly.

> Crust:
>
> 4½ teaspoons quick rising yeast
>
> 1 cup warm rice milk
>
> 1½ tablespoon olive oil
>
> 1 tablespoon maple syrup
>
> ¼ teaspoon salt
>
> 1 egg
>
> 2 cups rice flour
>
> 1 cup gluten-free flour mix (see below)
>
> 2 teaspoons xanthan gum
>
> 2 teaspoons GF Italian seasoning (optional)

Preheat oven to 350°F. In a mixer bowl, sprinkle yeast on top of warm rice milk. Let sit until the yeast foams (about 5 minutes). In another bowl, whisk together rice flour, gluten-free flour mix, xanthan gum and Italian seasoning (if being used). After the yeast/rice milk mixture has foamed, add olive oil, maple syrup, salt, and egg. Blend well. Add the dry ingredients to the wet. Using the paddle attachment of your mixer, beat ingredients well to form the dough. It should be close to ball form when ready. Turn dough onto a surface floured with gluten-free flour mix. Knead for a couple of minutes until dough feels smooth and is not as tacky to the touch. Divide dough in half. Roll or pat out two 12" circles. Place onto pizza pan or cookie sheet. Top with your favorite toppings. Drizzle mock pizza cheese (see below) over toppings, if desired.

Bake at 350°F preheated oven for 25–30 minutes.

MOCK PIZZA CHEESE

2 tablespoons GF/CF nutritional yeast powder (or 1 tablespoon nutritional yeast flakes)

2 tablespoons tapioca starch

½ teaspoon salt

¼ teaspoon garlic powder

1 cup water

1 tablespoon vegetable oil

1 teaspoon GF/CF prepared mustard

Whisk nutritional yeast, tapioca starch, salt, garlic powder, and water in a small saucepan. Cook over medium heat, whisking constantly, until thickened. Turn off heat. Whisk in vegetable oil and prepared mustard. Drizzle over pizza toppings while still warm before baking pizza. Enough for two 12" pizzas.

GF/CF CAKE

What is a party or birthday without cake! Light in texture and lightly sweetened, this cake is delicious with Maple Marshmallow Fluff Frosting. (see below)

¼ cup vegetable oil

⅔ cup maple syrup

1 egg

½ tablespoon GF vanilla flavor

1¾ cups GF flour mix (see below)

½ teaspoon xanthan gum

1 teaspoon baking soda

1 teaspoon baking powder

¼ teaspoon salt

Preheat oven to 350°F. Grease an 8" round cake pan. Sprinkle a bit of a GF flour of your choice in the pan and turn the pan so the flour coats the grease in the pan. Tap out excess flour. In a blender add oil, maple syrup, egg, and vanilla flavoring. Blend on high until well mixed. In a mixing bowl, whisk together GF flour mix, xanthan gum, baking soda, baking powder, and salt. Pour wet ingredients into bowl and stir just until well combined. Pour cake batter into prepared pan.

Bake in preheated oven for 25–30 minutes. Cake will be finished when a cake tester comes out clean. Do not over-bake as this will cause gluten-free bakery items to dry out faster. Cool 10 minutes in pan then remove to a cooling rack, if desired. Frost cake after cake has completely cooled.

MAPLE MARSHMALLOW FLUFF FROSTING

This is similar to Seven Minute Frosting, but without the refined sugar.

1 cup maple syrup

2 egg whites (you may use dry egg white powder reconstituted to equal 2 egg whites)

pinch of salt

In saucepan with a candy thermometer attached, whisk the maple syrup over medium to medium-high heat until syrup reaches 115°F. Turn off heat. In a mixer, whip egg whites and salt with whisk attachment until soft peaks form. With mixer running on low speed, slowly drizzle hot maple syrup into the egg whites. Whip on high until stiff peaks form. You may add food coloring now, if desired. Frost cake immediately, swirling icing into peaks all over the cake. Leave as is or sprinkle with GF sprinkles or crushed freeze-dried fruits (such as strawberries, apricots, or blueberries) for color before frosting sets.

GLUTEN-FREE FLOUR MIX

There are many different GF flour mixes and formulas out there. Please experiment to find the taste and texture your family enjoys. Below is a mix that does not include bean or corn, for those sensitive to those flours.

> 4 cups rice flour (brown, white, or a combination)
>
> 1 ⅓ cups potato starch
>
> ⅔ cup tapioca flour

You may use one cup of GF flour mix to replace a cup of wheat flour in your recipes. Be sure to add xanthan gum to your recipes also in the following amounts:

> Breads: ¾ teaspoon per cup of GF flour
>
> Cakes: ½ teaspoon per cup of GF flour
>
> Cookies: ¼ teaspoon per cup of GF flour

FLOURLESS NUTBUTTER COOKIES

If you can tolerate nuts, these are easy for the kids to help with.

> 2 cups natural peanut butter or nutbutter of your choice, such as almond
>
> 2 cups granulated sugar cane juice
>
> 2 eggs
>
> 1 teaspoon GF vanilla flavor

Preheat oven to 350°F. Cream nutbutter and granulated sugar cane juice well. Beat in eggs and vanilla. Drop by teaspoons onto a cookie sheet. Bake for 8–10 minutes until set. Let cool for a couple of minutes on pan before moving to cooling rack.

GUACAMOLE

Delicious with GF tortilla chips!!

> 2 ripe avocados
>
> 1½ tablespoon lemon or lime juice
>
> 1½ tablespoons minced sweet onion

½ teaspoon salt

1½ tablespoons olive oil

Cut avocados in half. Remove seeds. Scoop out the avocado pulp and put into a bowl. Coarsely mash avocado with a fork. Stir in lemon juice, minced onion, salt and olive oil. Cover bowl and chill for one hour.

OVEN FRIES

Easy to make, cheap, and healthier than store-bought. I find the kids are always impressed when I can make something they think can only come from the store. Replace one of the potatoes with a sweet potato or blue potato for a different and colorful taste treat. Add your favorite herbs and spices for seasoned fries.

4 potatoes

2½ tablespoons vegetable oil of choice

salt and pepper to taste

Preheat oven to 400°F. Lightly oil a medium jelly roll pan (baking tray). Slice potato into quarter inch strips and toss with oil. An easy way to do this is to put the oil and potato strips into a plastic bag. Seal bag and shake until potato strips are coated with oil. Put potato strips on pan in a single layer. Do not overlap. Bake for 25–30 minutes in oven. Turn the french fries over halfway through cooking time. When golden and crisp, season with salt and pepper to taste.

Serve with fruit-sweetened GF ketchup and GF honey mustard. You may also sprinkle with balsamic or cider vinegar for vinegar chips.

To drink

JUICE

Juice and sparkling mineral water

Chocolate or carob rice milk

Smoothie shakes

Peach Smoothie Shake

2 frozen bananas, cut in chunks

½ cup fresh or canned peaches, with juice

2 tablespoons fruit juice sweetened peach jam or preserves

¼ to ½ cup rice milk

In the order listed, place ingredients into blender. Add lid. Blend on high until smooth, adding more rice milk if needed.

To play with

GF PLAY DOUGH

Most play dough contains gluten, which gets under nails and is very difficult to completely wash off when it is time to eat, leading to gluten exposure. If you are looking for a purchased option, Crayola Model Magic and a play dough mix from Miss Roben's Grocery are currently available and gluten-free.

1 cup GF flour mix (see above)

½ cup salt

2 teaspoons cream of tartar

1 cup water

1 teaspoon cooking oil

food coloring

Whisk ingredients in a saucepan. Cook over medium heat stirring constantly until mixture thickens and forms a ball. Put play dough on a surface dusted with GF flour mix and knead until smooth when cooled to a touchable temperature. Store in plastic bag or container after play dough completely cools.

You can view Angela's website at www.angelaskitchen.com

GF/CF Foods

The Gluten Free Pantry
http://www.glutenfreemall.com

Miss Roben's: Your Allergy Grocer
(free recipes)
http://www.missroben.com

The Gluten Free Kitchen
(has children's corner and free recipes)
http://gfkitchen.server101.com

The Gluten-Free Mall
http://www.glutenfreemall.com

Gluten Solutions
http://www.glutensolutions.com/

The Allergy Free Food Shop
http://www.dietaryneedsdirect.co.uk

The Gluten-Free Food Vendor Directory
http://www.gfmall.com

Kinnikinnick Foods
http://www.kinnikinnick.com

Lifestyle Health Care
http://www.glutenfree.com.uk

Schaer
http://www.schaer.com

Raymond-Hadley Corporation
http://www.raymondhadley.com

GF/CF Books

Jackson, L. (2001) *A User Guide to the GF/CF Diet for Autism, Asperger Syndrome and AD/HD*. London: Jessica Kingsley Publishers.

Legge, B. (2001) *Can't Eat, Won't Eat: Dietary Difficulties and Autistic Spectrum Disorders*. London: Jessica Kingsley Publishers.

Le Breton, M. (2001) *Diet Intervention and Autism: Implementing the Gluten Free and Casein Free Diet for Autistic Children and Adults – A Practical Guide for Parents*. London: Jessica Kingsley Publishers.

Le Breton, M. (2002) *The AiA Gluten and Dairy Free Cookbook*. London: Jessica Kingsley Publishers.

Lewis, L. (1999) *Special Diets for Special Kids: Understanding and Implementing Special Diets to Aid in the Treatment of Autism and Related Developmental Disorders*. Arlington, TX: Future Horizons.

Helpful Organizations

Allergy Alert Bracelets
www.medicalert.org

Allergy Associates of LaCrosse
www.allergy-solutions.com

Autism-Diet E-Mail Support Group
www.yahoogroups.com/group/Autism-Diet

Autism Europe
http://osiris.sunderland.ac.uk/autism/eur.html

Allergy Induced Autism (AiA)
http://www.autismdiet.co.uk/top.htm

Autism Network for Dietary Intervention
www.AutismNDI.com
(support for families using GF/CF diets for autism)

Autism Research Unit, School of Health Science Sunderland, UK
http://osiris.sunderland.ac.uk/autism/

Autism UK web Site
http://www.autism-uk.ed.ac.uk/

Developmental Delay Resources (DDR)
http://www.devdelay.org/
(numerous resources)

GFCF Autism Diet Therapy
http://www.gfcfdiet.com
(excellent resource)

Gluten Intolerance Group
http://www.gluten.net

National Autistic Society (UK)
htpp://www.nas.org.uk/

Miss Roben's: Your Allergy Grocer

http://www.missroben.com

(online catalog and free recipes)

Public Autism Awareness

http://www.paains.org.uk/index.html

(up-to-the-minute autism news from around the world)

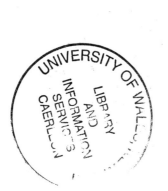